TEEN GUIDE TO MENTAL HEALTH

TEEN GUIDE: HELPING SOMEONE IN CRISIS

by Philip Wolny

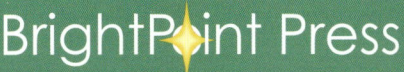

San Diego, CA

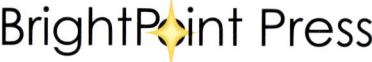

© 2026 BrightPoint Press
an imprint of ReferencePoint Press, Inc.
Printed in the United States

For more information, contact:
BrightPoint Press
PO Box 27779
San Diego, CA 92198
www.BrightPointPress.com

ALL RIGHTS RESERVED.

No part of this work covered by the copyright hereon may be reproduced or used in any form or by any means—graphic, electronic, or mechanical, including photocopying, recording, taping, web distribution, or information storage retrieval systems—without the written permission of the publisher.

Content Consultant: Raymond Blanchard, PhD, LMHC-D, NCC, CCMHC, Assistant Professor and Clinical Coordinator of Clinical Mental Health Counseling, Molloy University

---

LIBRARY OF CONGRESS CATALOGING-IN-PUBLICATION DATA

Names: Wolny, Philip author
Title: Teen guide: helping someone in crisis / by Philip Wolny.
Other titles: Helping someone in crisis
Description: San Diego, CA: ReferencePoint Press, [2026] | Series: Teen guide to mental health | Includes bibliographical references and index. | Audience: Grades 7–9
Identifiers: LCCN 2025002077 (print) | LCCN 2025002078 (eBook) | ISBN 9781678211448 (hardcover) | ISBN 9781678211455 (eBook)
Subjects: LCSH: Teenagers--Mental health--Juvenile literature | Mentally ill teenagers--Care--Juvenile literature | Crisis intervention (Mental health services)--Juvenile literature
Classification: LCC RJ499 .W565 2026 (print) | LCC RJ499 (eBook) | DDC 618.92/89--dc23/eng/20250324
LC record available at https://lccn.loc.gov/2025002077
LC eBook record available at https://lccn.loc.gov/2025002078

CONTENTS

CONTENT WARNING: THIS BOOK DESCRIBES SUICIDE AND SUICIDAL THOUGHTS, WHICH MAY BE TRIGGERING TO SOME READERS.

AT A GLANCE   4

INTRODUCTION   6
FINDING WAYS TO HELP

CHAPTER ONE   12
IDENTIFYING A MENTAL HEALTH CRISIS

CHAPTER TWO   28
ENGAGING SOMEONE IN CRISIS

CHAPTER THREE   42
LONG-TERM HELP AND HEALING

Glossary	58
Source Notes	59
For Further Research	60
Index	62
Image Credits	63
About the Author	64

AT A GLANCE

- A mental health crisis is when a person experiences behaviors or symptoms that can lead them to hurt themselves or others.

- Mental health crises may be caused by many factors, including health conditions, substance abuse, discrimination, financial status, racism, and bullying.

- Warning signs of a crisis may include negative language, changes in behavior, loss of interest in hobbies, self-harm, or aggression.

- Watching and listening are key to figuring out whether someone is in crisis. People in crisis may try to hide their problems from others.

- When helping someone in crisis, people should stay calm, respect the person and their privacy, and be present for the person.

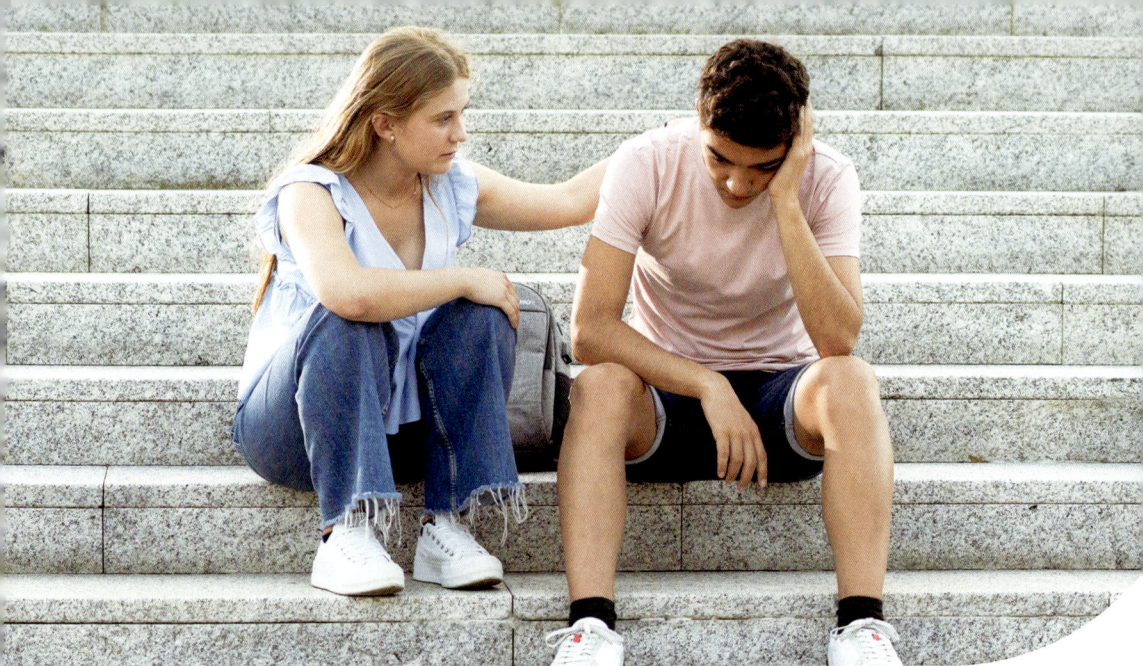

- If a crisis reaches a tipping point, teens should reach out to a trusted adult or authority figure for help. A trusted adult may be a parent, relative, teacher, or mental health professional.

- Mental health resources are available online and in person. Walk-in clinics, hospital emergency room visits, and crisis hotlines are options for those who cannot wait for a therapy appointment.

- Long-term help and healing are often needed to prevent future mental health crises. Friends, family, and communities can provide support for a person dealing with a crisis.

INTRODUCTION

FINDING WAYS TO HELP

Azin Anees was a high schooler from San Jose, California. In 2021, she was shocked to learn that her community had a serious problem. The suicide rate was five times higher than the US national average. Azin decided to act. She started volunteering for Samaritans. Samaritans is an organization working to prevent suicide. It also helps people who have lost someone to suicide.

In 2023, suicide was the second-leading cause of death among teens and young adults.

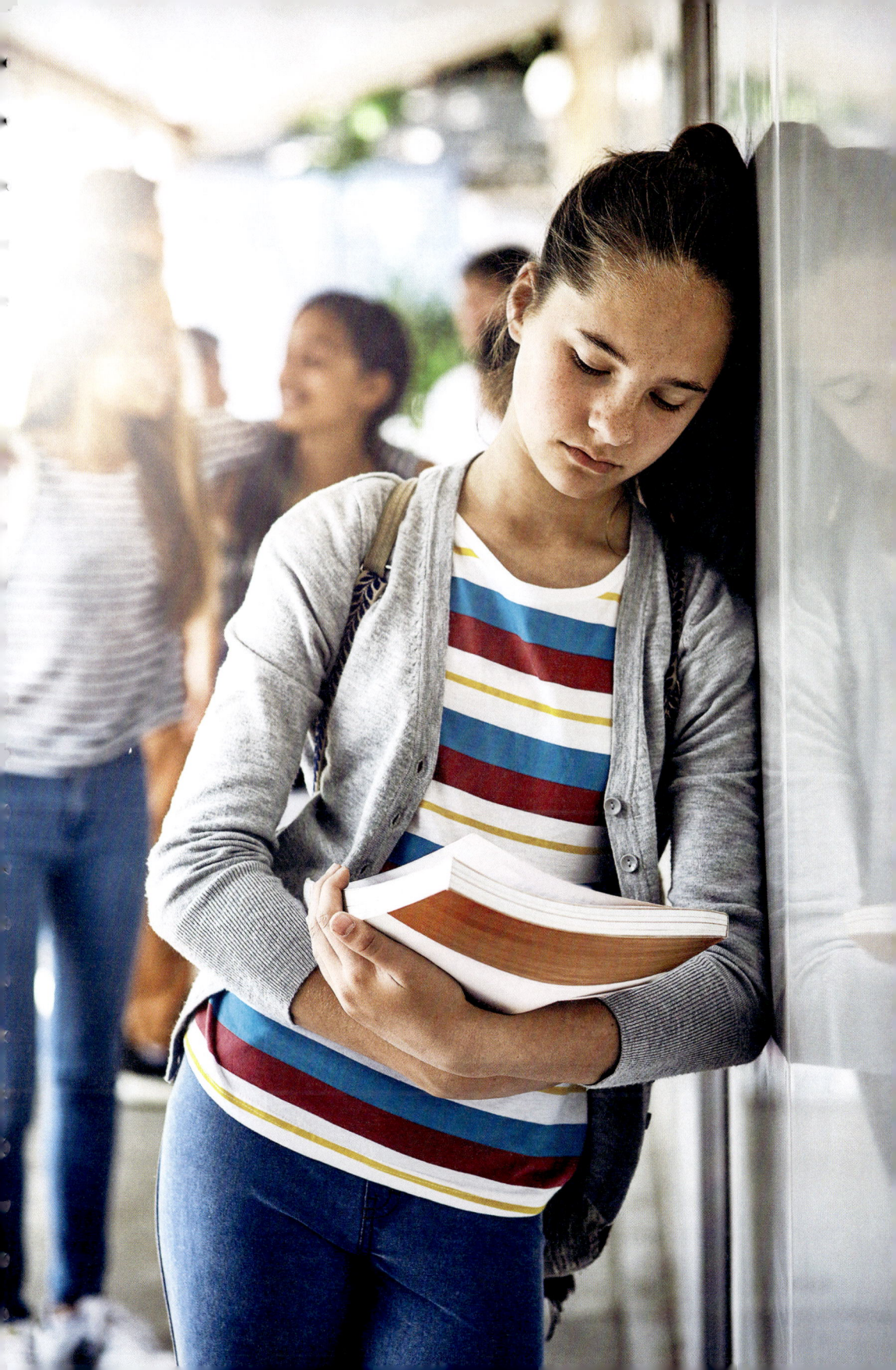

Azin volunteered on the 24/7 crisis hotline. The hotline provides help to those with mental health issues. People can talk to volunteers. This can be done through phone calls or texts.

Azin trained for how to talk to those in crisis. She provided help for hundreds of people. "By volunteering on the helpline, I am able to provide a safe and nonjudgmental listening ear for callers and texters," she said.[1]

But Azin did not stop there. Her experience at Samaritans inspired her own project. She launched Let's Talk Mental Health. It helped teens in need at her high school. The project spread mental health awareness as well. Azin also started the Let's Talk Mental Health podcast to reach

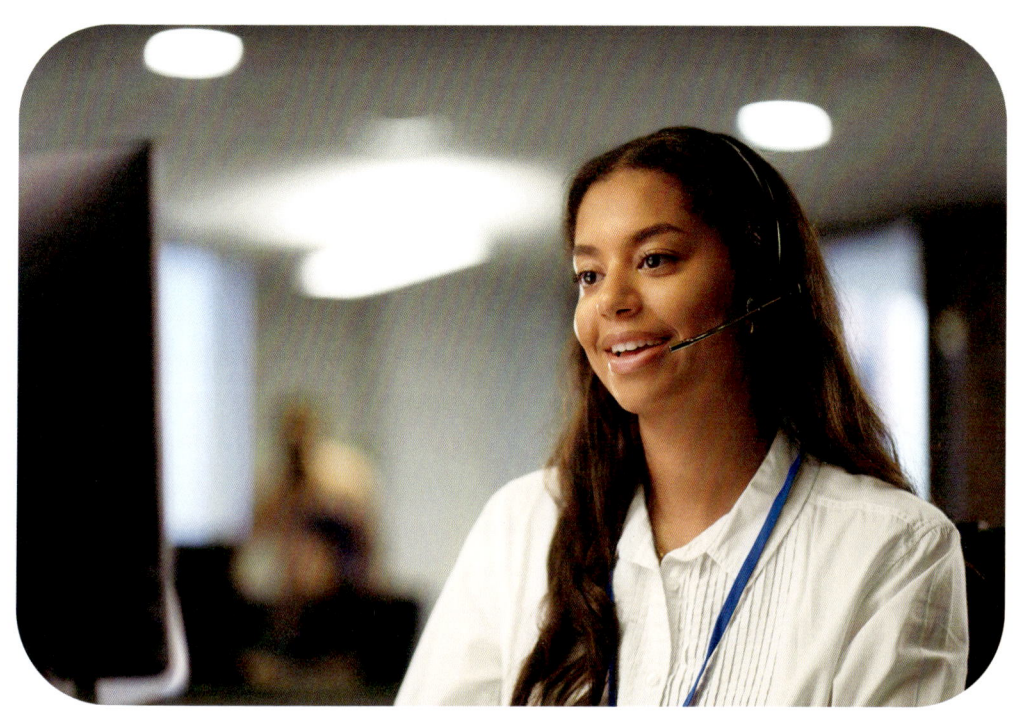

Some teen crisis hotlines require volunteers to be at least 15 years old.

more people. Through Let's Talk Mental Health, Azin was able to help those in crisis.

HELP AND SUPPORT

Azin is just one of many people helping those who struggle with mental health. Mental health issues have risen globally since 2010. Many factors have affected people's mental health. These include

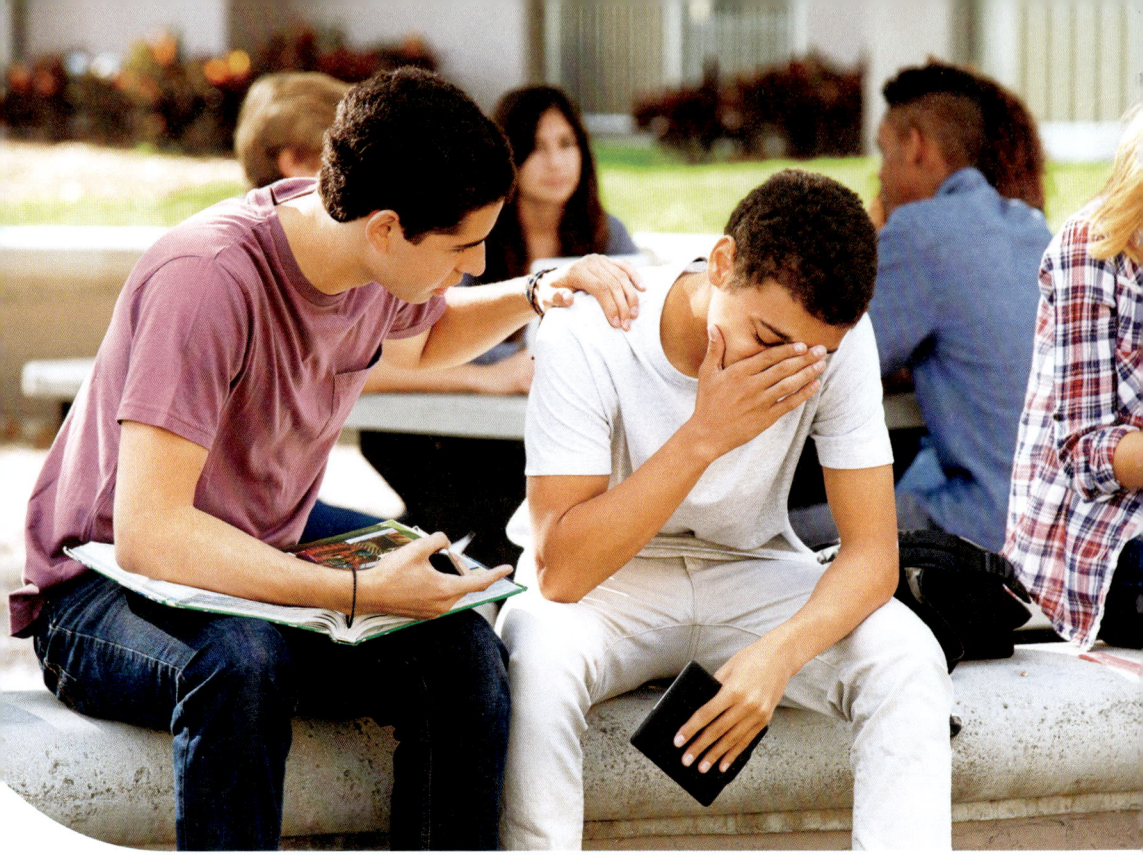

Mental health struggles can affect many aspects of a person's life.

substance abuse, bullying, and other health issues. Some people may have trouble finding the support they need. Without support, a person could be pushed to their limit. They may experience a mental health crisis.

Millions of people with mental health issues are at risk of crises. But friends, family, and community members can help. They can pay attention to the signs. They can learn how to talk to those in crisis. And they can connect people to mental health resources. Anyone can find ways to support and help those in crisis.

Many people and organizations around the United States work to support teens dealing with mental health crises.

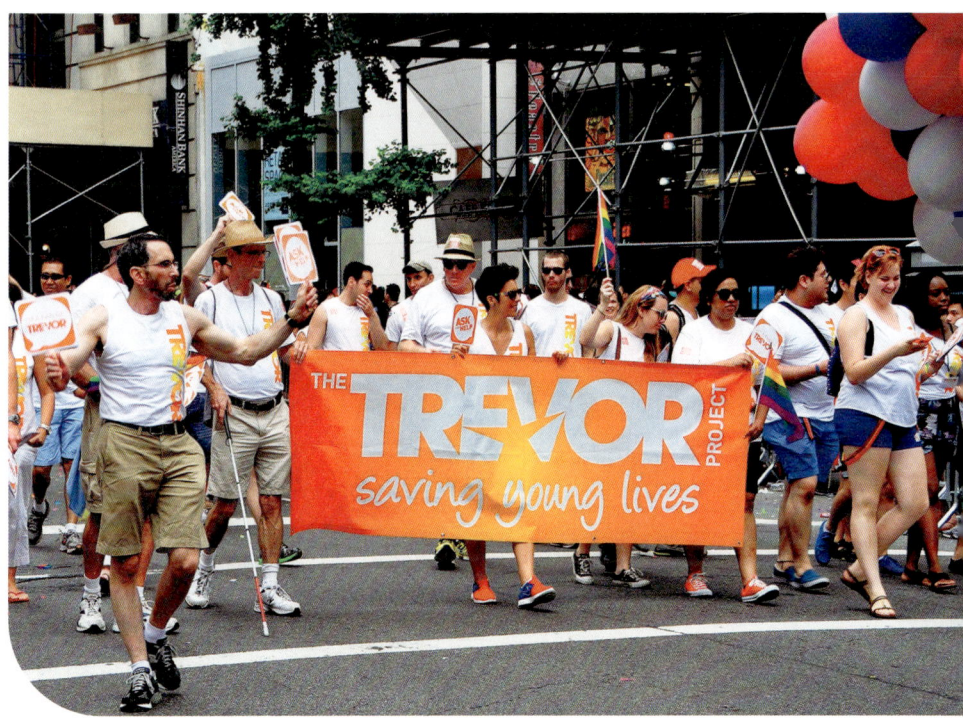

CHAPTER ONE

IDENTIFYING A MENTAL HEALTH CRISIS

Mental health has been a topic of focus for many years. Awareness of mental health issues grew in the early 2000s. Teenagers are especially vulnerable to mental health challenges. They experience changes to their bodies and minds. They juggle school, athletics, jobs, and other activities. They have relationships with family, friends, and classmates. And many young people use social media.

Teens can feel pressured to maintain grades, activities, and relationships.

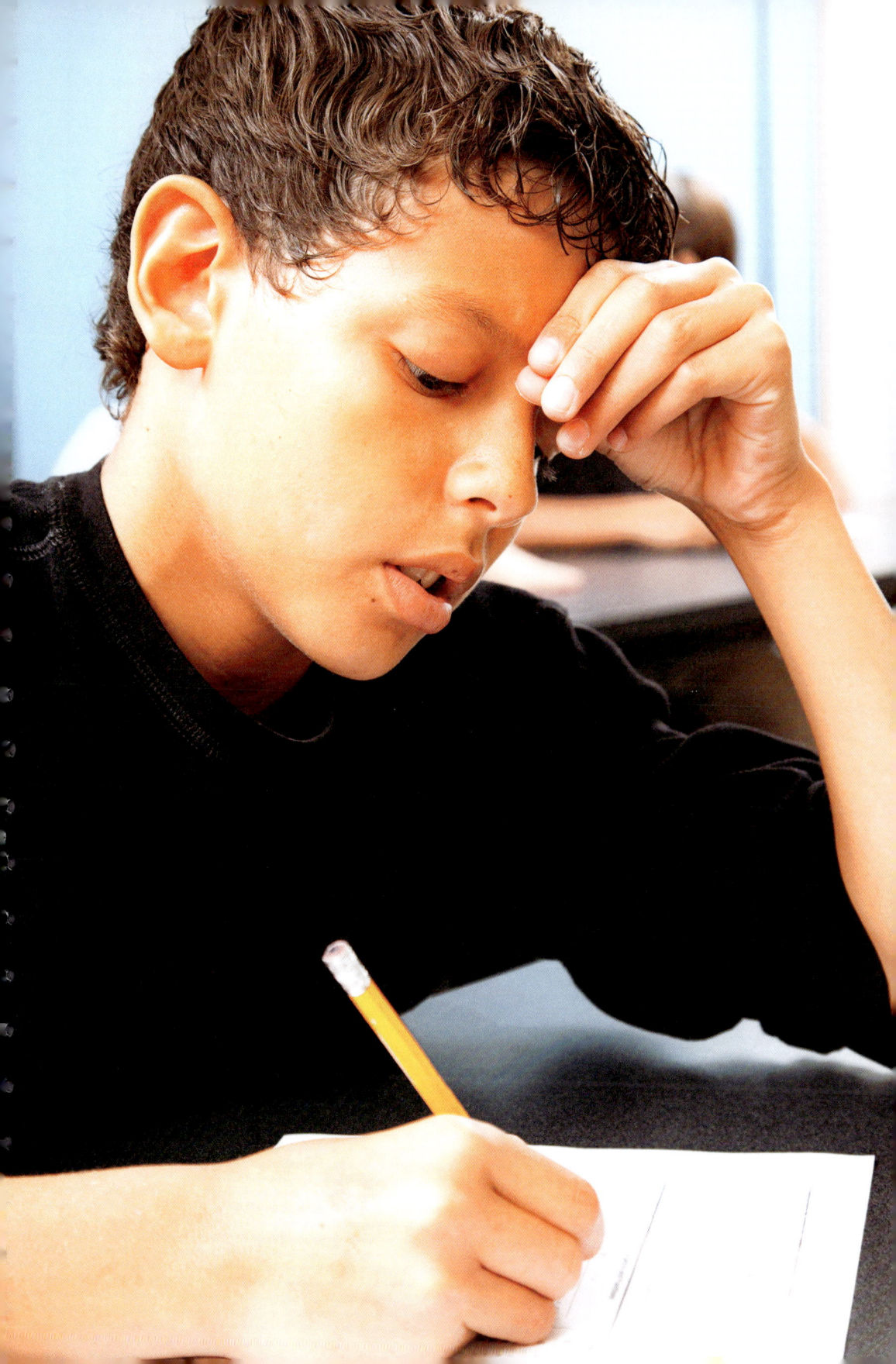

Balancing these factors can be stressful. Sometimes, teens experience mental health issues. These may include depression and anxiety. Without help, mental health issues can spiral into a crisis. This is

Teens may hide their mental health struggles from friends and family members.

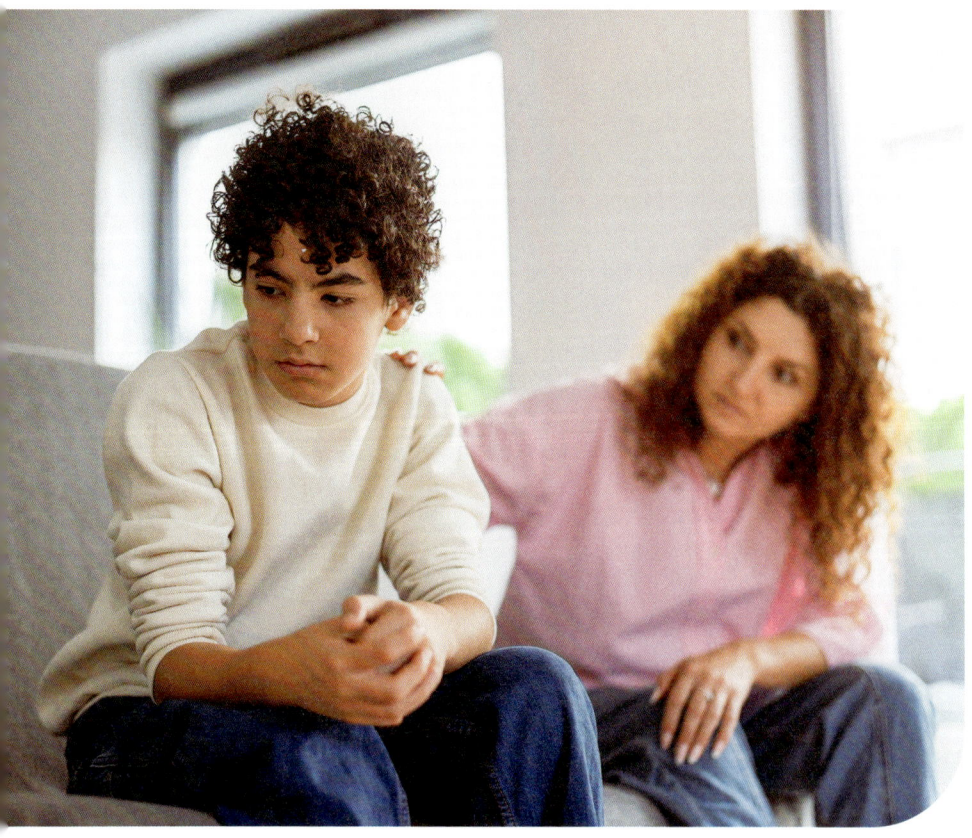

when a person experiences behaviors or symptoms that may lead them to hurt themselves or others. A crisis may cause a person to be less interested in the things they once enjoyed. Someone in crisis may also not be able to take care of themselves properly. There are many types of mental health crises.

A WIDESPREAD PROBLEM

Today, teenagers deal with many pressures. They may be pressured to fit in with peers. Or they may be affected by global issues. The COVID-19 pandemic is one example. Lockdowns and other measures began in 2020. These caused teens around the world to feel isolated. Youth mental illness increased during that time.

According to the National Alliance on Mental Illness (NAMI), one in six people between the ages of 6 and 17 deal with a mental health disorder each year. Some youth experience depression. Others deal with anxiety. People with bipolar disorder can have extreme changes in emotion and energy. Some teens have other mental health disorders or several disorders.

UNDER PRESSURE

Being a teenager can be difficult. Teens face challenges daily. They may feel pressure to be high achievers in school and in sports. They may not take time to relax or focus on self-care. Some teenagers also deal with bullying or isolation. These issues may occur in person or online.

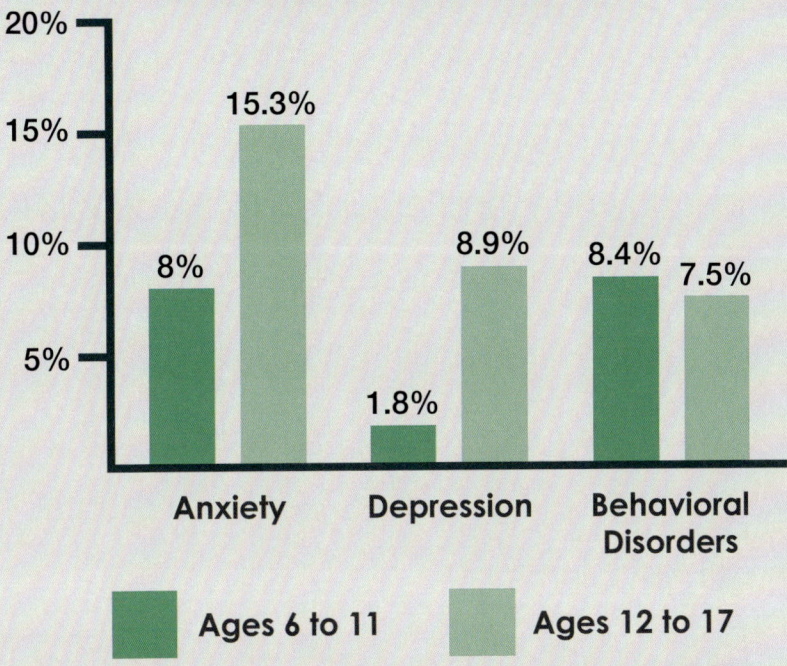

Source: "Data and Statistics on Children's Mental Health," *Children's Mental Health*, August 19, 2024. www.cdc.gov.

According to Children's Mental Health, anxiety, depression, and behavioral disorders are the most common mental health conditions diagnosed in children and teens.

Online bullying and other negative behaviors can happen around the clock.

Challenges at home also affect mental health. Mental or physical abuse is harmful. Parents or relatives may have substance abuse issues. Or they may deal with their own mental health problems. Unemployment and other family hardships may cause teens stress. Kids in families dealing with financial struggles are at a higher risk for mental health issues. Even youth who seem fine may deal with mental health problems.

Marginalized Groups

Mental health issues are often higher for teens in minority and **marginalized** groups. These groups also have trouble finding support. More than 50 percent of LGBTQ+ teens suffer from mental health problems. And 56 percent said they wanted mental health care but could not get it. One organization that provides mental health support is the Trevor Project. It focuses on suicide prevention for young people in the LGBTQ+ community.

Some teens face discrimination. This is when people are treated badly because of their race, ethnicity, or religion. Others experience gender or sexual orientation discrimination. Peers may make fun of a person's weight. Anxiety about self-image can lead to serious issues, such as an eating disorder. All these pressures build up. They may affect teens in harmful ways.

TRIGGERING A CRISIS

A mental health crisis can be triggered by many things. Minor issues or events can escalate into major problems. It could be an argument with family or friends. A relationship breakup may cause a person to feel sad or depressed. So can the deaths of loved ones. Both **traumatic** events and everyday setbacks can trigger crises. This might cause a person to become a danger to themselves or others.

Physical health problems affect mental health as well. When Sierra was in eighth grade, she got very sick. The illness gave her headaches. It also made her tired. One year later, Sierra started struggling with anxiety. By tenth grade, she had developed depression. "I didn't recognize my suffering was depression until the day I picked up a razor, seeing it as an escape," said Sierra. "I cut my right arm, just a little bit."[2]

This led her to cut herself more. Eventually, Sierra realized she needed help. She wrote a letter to her parents about her struggles. They rushed her to the hospital. Sierra spent time in therapy. Years of

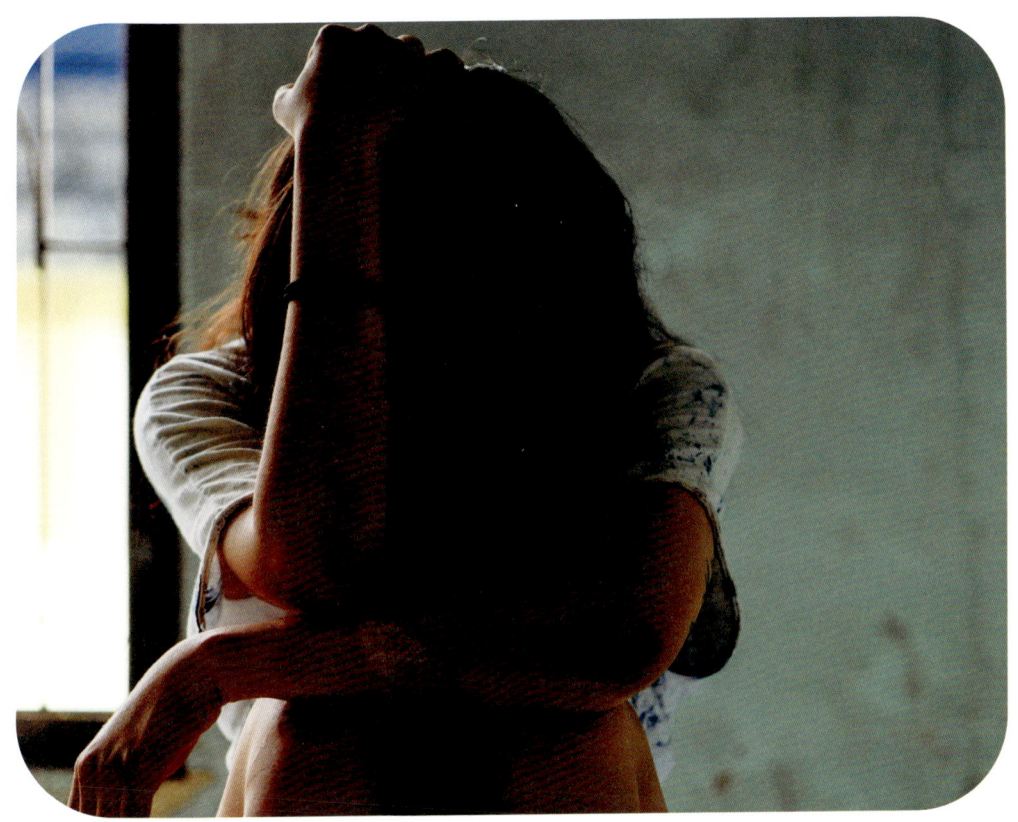

Cutting is the most common method of self-harm.

treatment helped her deal with her anxiety and depression. But her struggles began with a physical health problem.

WARNING SIGNS

Teens are often best at understanding others their age. Peers may share their experiences and problems with one another. Adults in teens' lives might be busy, absent, or distracted. Lisa Damour is a journalist for *The New York Times*. She writes about mental health issues. Damour wrote, "Teenagers are usually great supports for one another . . . often outside of adults' awareness."[3]

Friends are often the first to notice early warning signs of someone in crisis. These signs can vary from person to person. A friend could be absent from class for some time. Or a person's appearance might have changed. They may look sick. They could appear more tired than usual. Or they may have gained or lost weight quickly.

Someone in crisis may start behaving differently. Unusual behavior could be a symptom of a certain mental illness.

It could also be caused by alcohol or drug abuse. Some people deal with challenges by using drugs or alcohol. They may even abuse drugs that were prescribed for a health condition.

Some people with mental health struggles believe alcohol and drugs can help them deal with their issues.

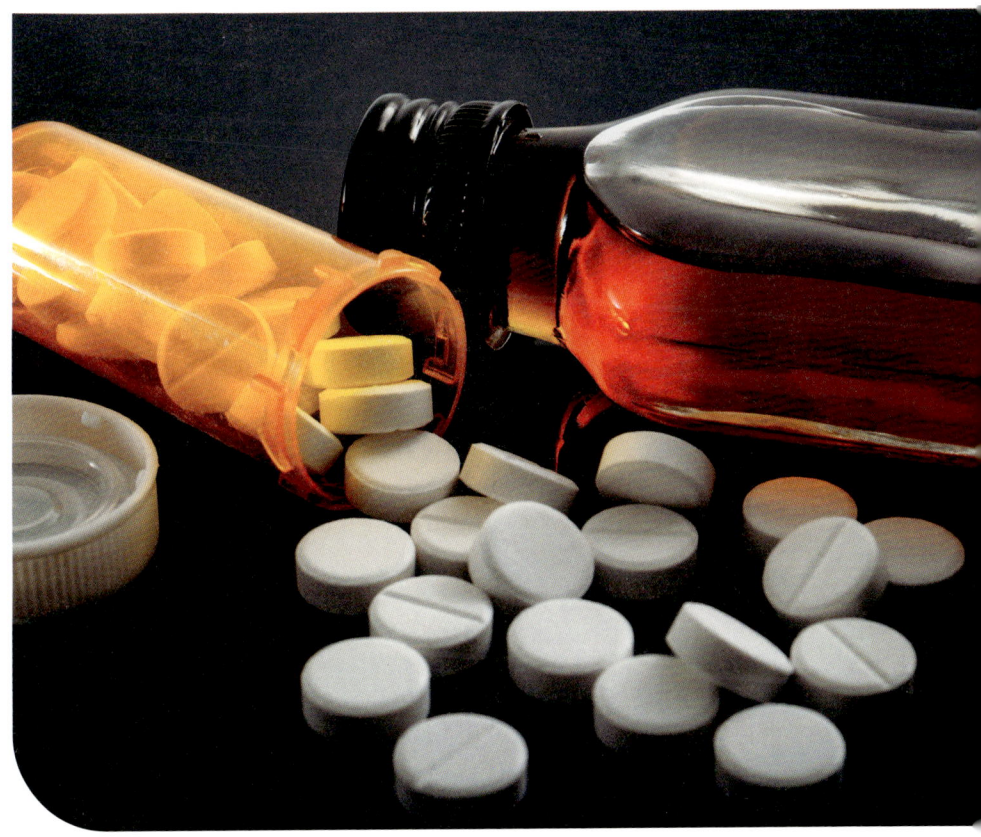

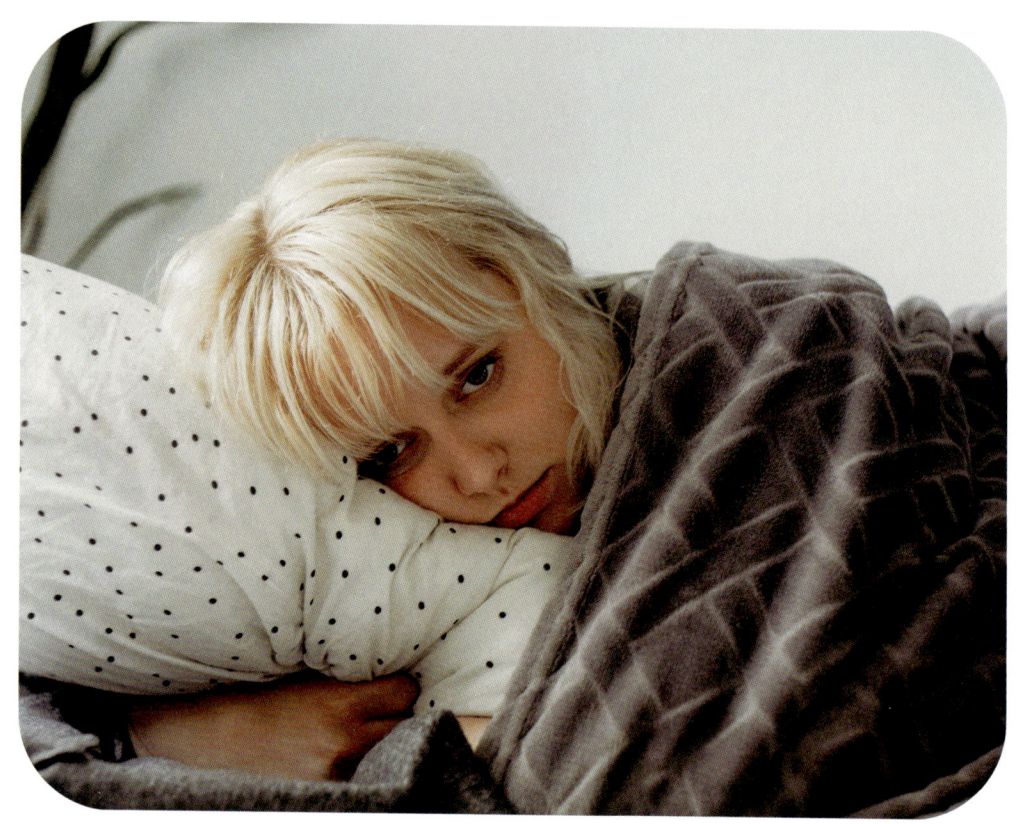

Sleeping all the time or not sleeping very much can both be signs that someone is experiencing a mental health crisis.

Someone dealing with a mental crisis may lose interest in things they used to enjoy. They may give up their favorite hobby or quit a team. Their energy levels might change. They may suddenly have a new set of friends. These friends may be negative influences on them or their mental state.

THINGS GET SERIOUS

Other warning signs of a mental health crisis are more serious. Cuts, bruises, or burns may be signs of self-harm. Explanations about the injuries might seem suspicious. The person may be trying to hide their crisis.

Another sign is a person not taking care of themselves. They may seem dirty or unwashed. They may not change their clothes regularly. A lack of self-care can signal that a person's mental health is suffering.

People in crisis may also have major mood swings. One minute they may be sad. The next they may become angry or aggressive. They might overreact to everyday problems or setbacks.

Negative language is another sign of a mental health crisis. Teens may tell friends that they are feeling sad or hopeless. They may say that they are worthless or no good. Some might question the point of living at all. A serious warning sign is if someone says they want to commit suicide.

Teens dealing with mental health crises may appear moodier than others their age.

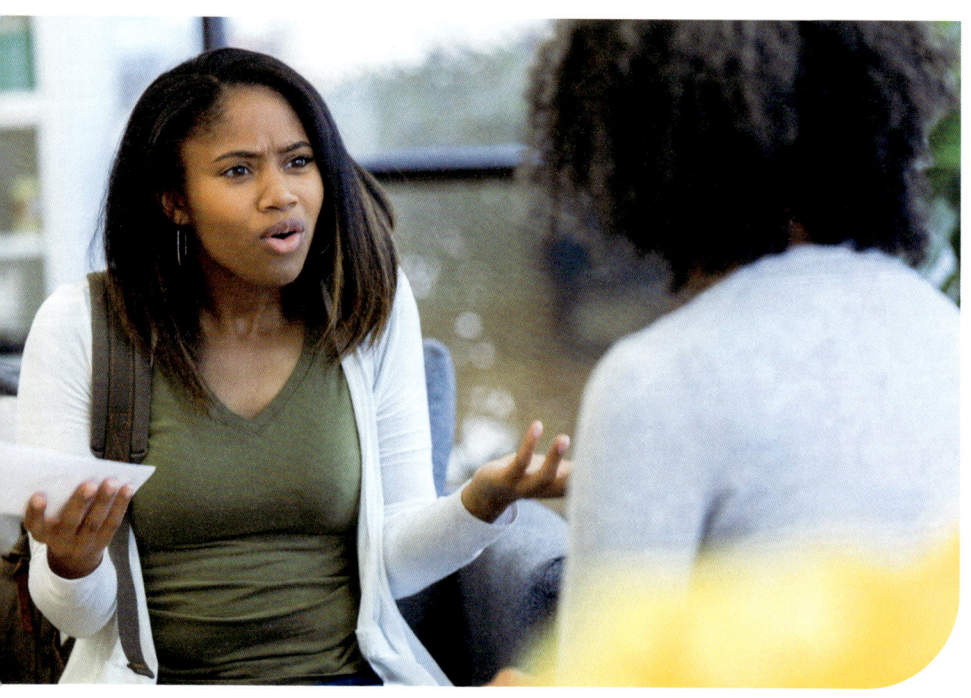

The friend might not intend to actually harm themselves. But they may not know another way to ask for help.

Some people do not feel comfortable asking for help directly. They may post their thoughts online. This could be another sign that they need help.

Episodes of rage or violence might also mean someone is in crisis. Teens under stress might have panic attacks. Hearing voices or having hallucinations can also be signs of a more serious mental health issue. Warning signs can be big or small. But once they are noticed, the next step is to take action to help the person in crisis.

CHAPTER TWO

ENGAGING SOMEONE IN CRISIS

Many people know someone who has faced mental health challenges. That person could be a classmate, best friend, parent, or sibling. However, people may not always get the support they need.

In 2023, almost 60 percent of kids who struggled with major depression reported not getting help. People who do not have support may feel helpless. They may believe suicide is their only option. Experts estimate

Many teens dealing with mental health struggles may feel as if they are alone.

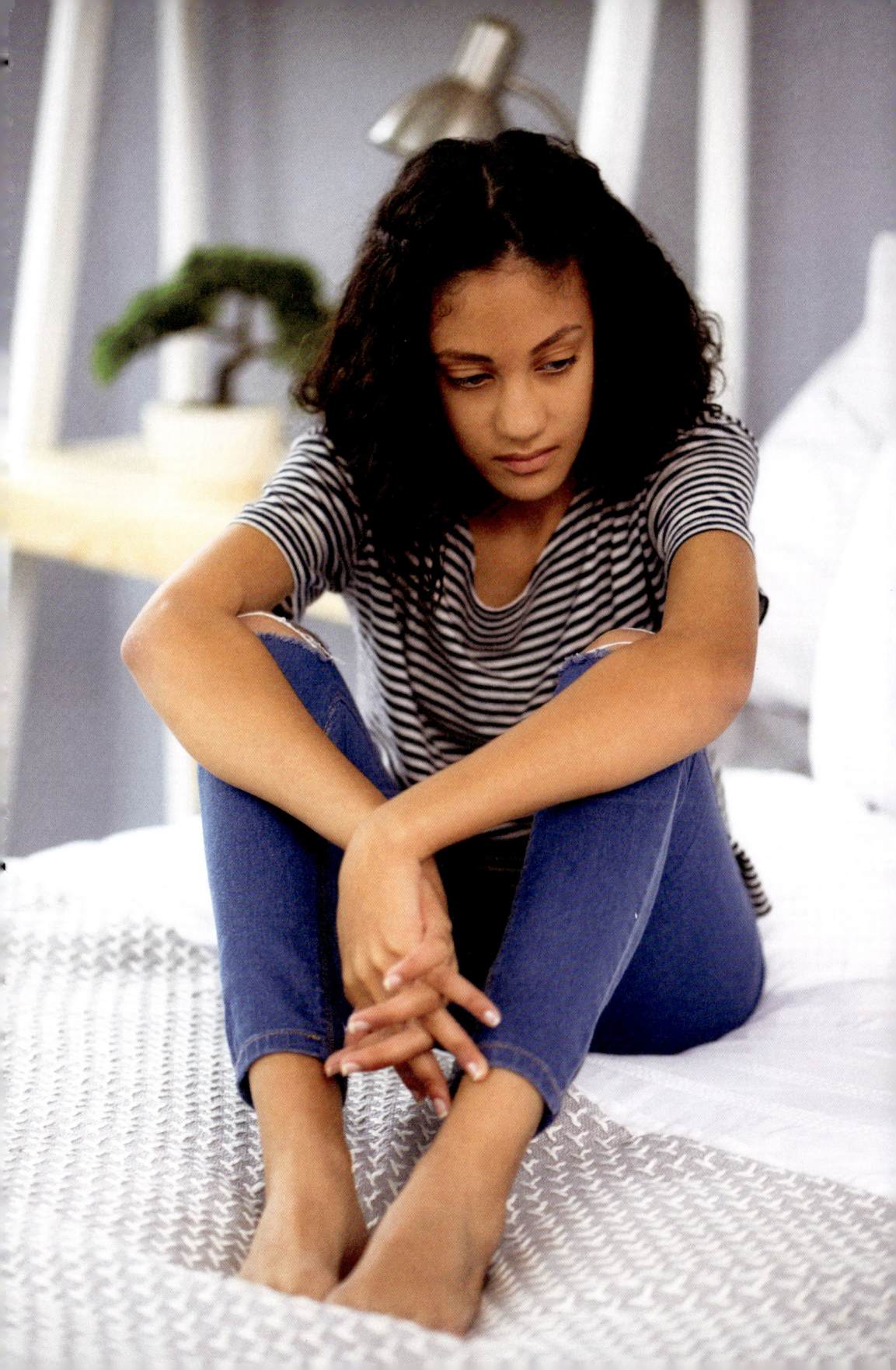

that teen suicide has risen by about 60 percent since 2010.

LEARNING TO LISTEN

People can help those in crisis in different ways. Watching and listening are important steps. These can be easier to do when the helper knows the person in crisis well. Some people can tell whether a friend or family member is acting out of character.

Sometimes, a direct approach is best. Questions such as "Are you okay?" or "How have things been for you lately?" can start a conversation. The conversation can happen in person. Or it can take place through text or social media messaging. People checking in on those in crisis should use a respectful and caring approach.

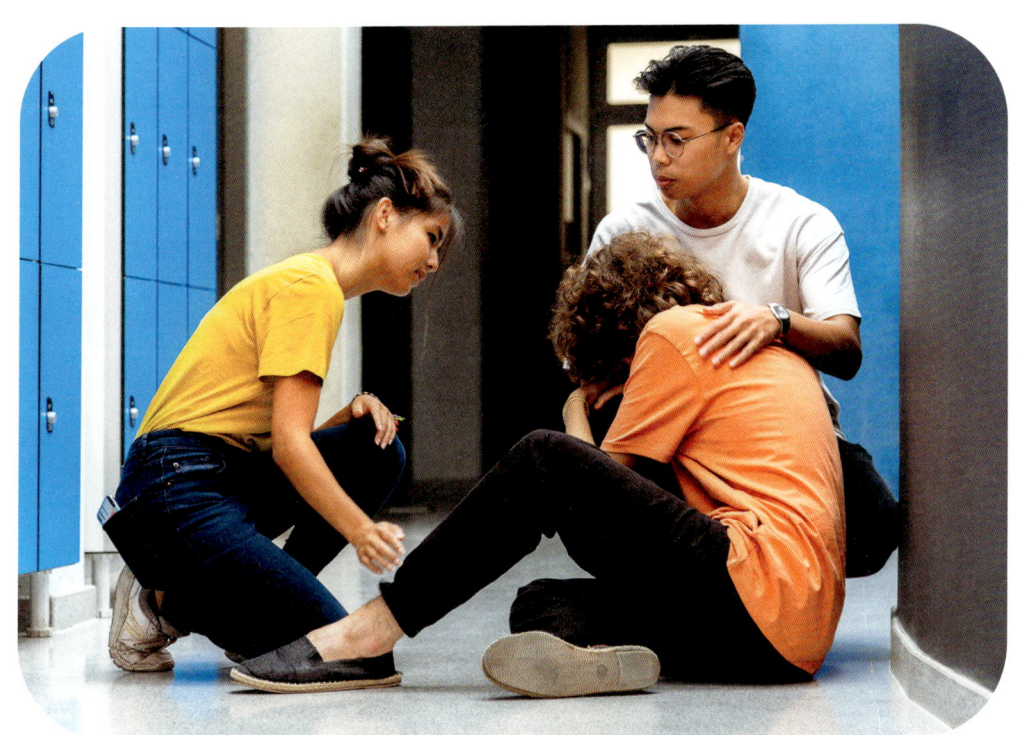

Asking open-ended questions is one way to help those in crisis talk about their feelings. Open-ended questions cannot be answered with just a yes or no.

Stephen Satterfield is from Fruita, Colorado. When he was a teenager, Stephen felt suicidal. He talked about how a best friend's call saved him. He said, "When I was ten minutes away from ending it all, my best friend Kyler called me . . . and we started talking about my problems. Kyler proved to me that people love me and care about me. Even though I didn't believe it at first, I'm happy I listened to what he said."[4]

In other cases, an indirect approach might work better. Inviting someone to just hang out can be a start. The concerned person can work their way up to asking

Someone in crisis may need a physical or emotional safe space to help them feel more comfortable talking about their mental health.

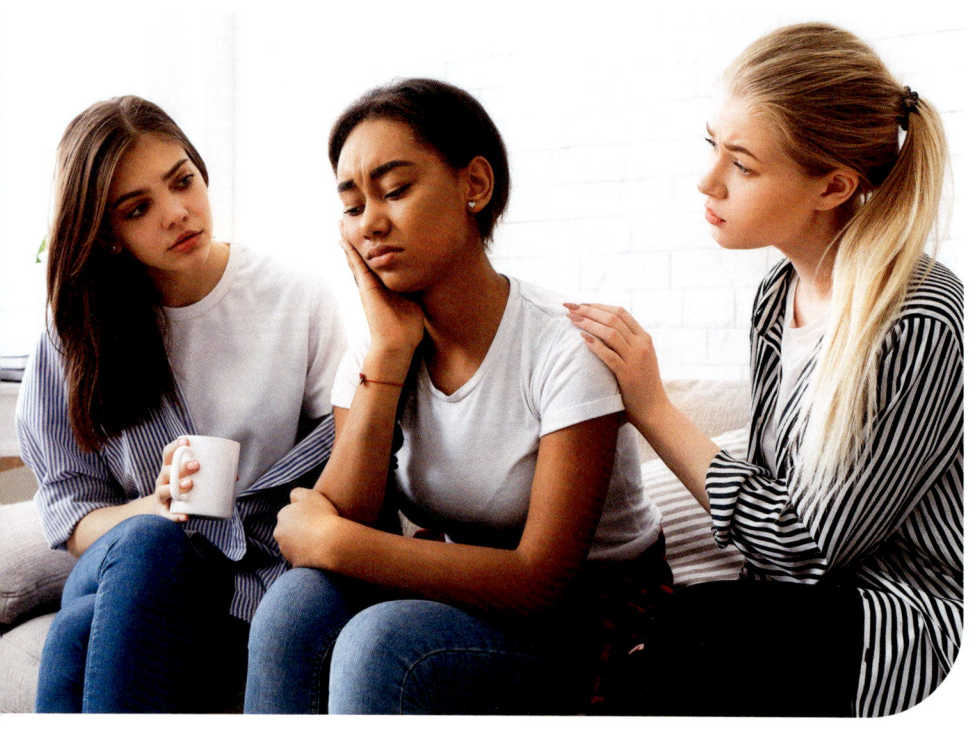

about the other person's mental health. People in crisis sometimes get anxious from too much attention. This may happen even if someone is trying to help.

Humor may also help someone in crisis to open up. The person might not want to think about their problems all the time. They may need some cheering up first. The person engaging must figure out whether humor is the right approach.

ENGAGING WITH PATIENCE AND RESPECT

Just showing up and being present can be enough for some people. This helps those in crisis know that someone cares. They will feel **validated**. They feel supported during a hard time.

People should be calm and respectful when engaging with a person in crisis. The person needs to know their feelings are valued. Their boundaries must be respected. The person might just need someone to be there for them. They also might not want to be told what to do. They may feel despair, anger, or a lack of control. Some people simply need to **vent** their feelings.

Psychologist Kenneth Carter discussed how helping requires patience. He wrote, "Sometimes you will be focused on wanting the other person to feel better or to take away their pain. . . . You may be ready to offer up a solution, but they may not be ready to hear one yet."[5] In such cases, the person in crisis may need to express

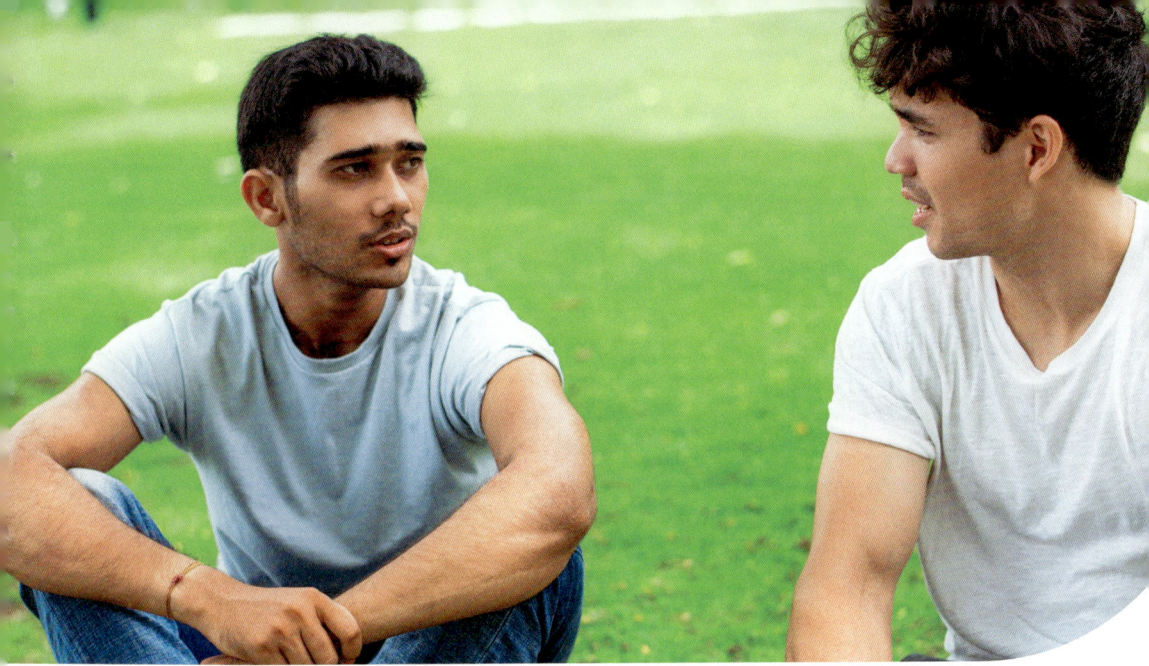

When helping someone in crisis, people should try to listen more than they talk. This allows those in crisis to feel heard.

their negative emotions. This is known as emotion-focused **coping**.

People who want to help should not make the situation about themselves. Telling someone in crisis that they will get over the situation can negatively affect them. Statements such as "I'm sorry this is happening" or "This must be so frustrating," are more helpful. These statements show **empathy**.

REACHING THE LIMIT

Some people in crisis might not want to be helped. They might be hitting a breaking point. They could feel scared about what they are experiencing.

Sometimes, people who are trying to help take on too much. They may even be trying to help multiple people through crises. Dealing with other people's troubles

Peer-to-Peer Help

The University of Michigan has a resource called the Peer-to-Peer Depression Awareness Program. This program offers peer counseling. It trains students to talk to one another about mental health. Many youths respond better to help from those their own age. The program has grown to more than fifty middle schools and high schools across the United States.

can be exhausting. Emotional exhaustion could be a sign of **burnout**. So can changes in sleeping patterns and anxiety. When a person's own mental health suffers, it is time to disengage and take a break.

APPROACHING A TRUSTED ADULT

Listening or giving advice might not always be enough. For example, a teenager may need to get a trusted adult involved. The adult may be a parent or guardian of the person in need. They could also be a teacher or counselor. Adults can provide resources that teens do not have easy access to.

Some teens may not want adults in their lives to know about their crisis. They may have good reasons for being secretive.

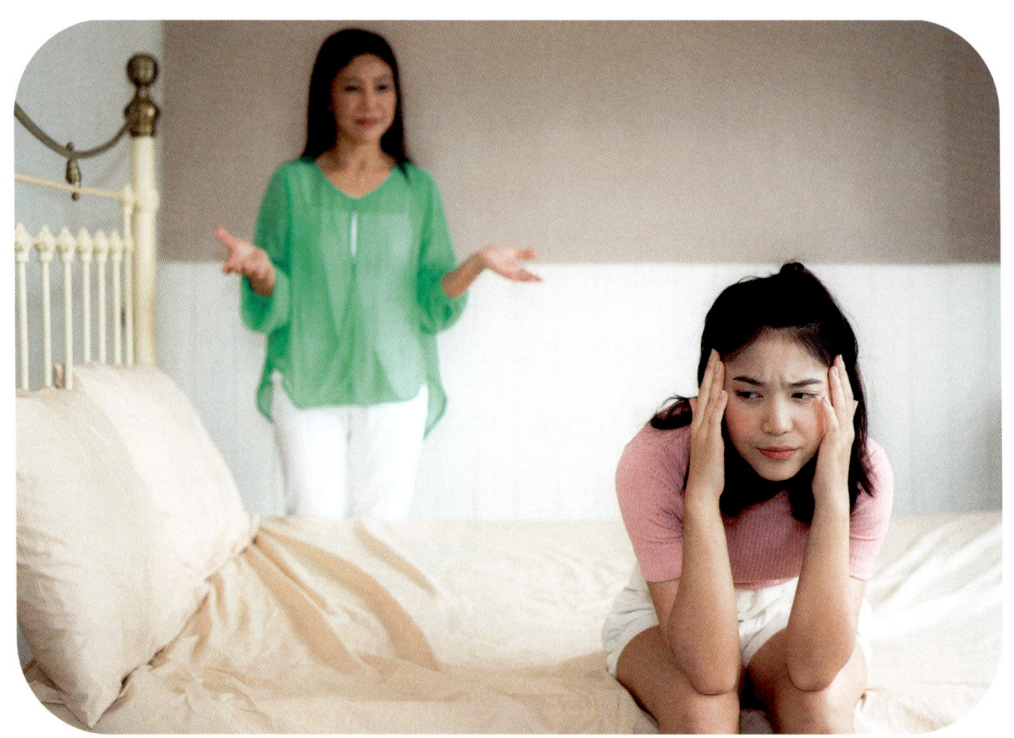

Parents can worsen their teen's mental health by being too overprotective, by being verbally abusive, or by not showing interest in their lives.

For example, the parent may be causing the crisis. Physical abuse, emotional abuse, or substance abuse can make home life hard. Telling the wrong person may lead to more abuse or neglect.

Lindsay Macchia is a psychologist. She explains how someone can help a troubled person without breaking their privacy.

She says, "There's a way to go about it without tattling. It's all about openness and honesty." Macchia suggests telling the person in crisis that it might be time to ask an adult for help. "This can be extremely tough, and of course you would want to preserve your friendship as best as you can. That being said, however, your friend's safety and well-being come first."[6]

Telling a person's parents or family is a first step. If that is not possible, other trusted adults can be approached. A teacher could be an option. Most schools have guidance counselors. Some even have therapists. These professionals are there to help. If a problem is serious, they know who to contact outside of the school for assistance. Sports coaches may be an option. Faith leaders might also be able to assist.

Some people in crisis might be in immediate danger to themselves or others. In that case, the best choice may be to call emergency services. This could mean calling for an ambulance.

School guidance counselors can provide support to teens who may be in crisis.

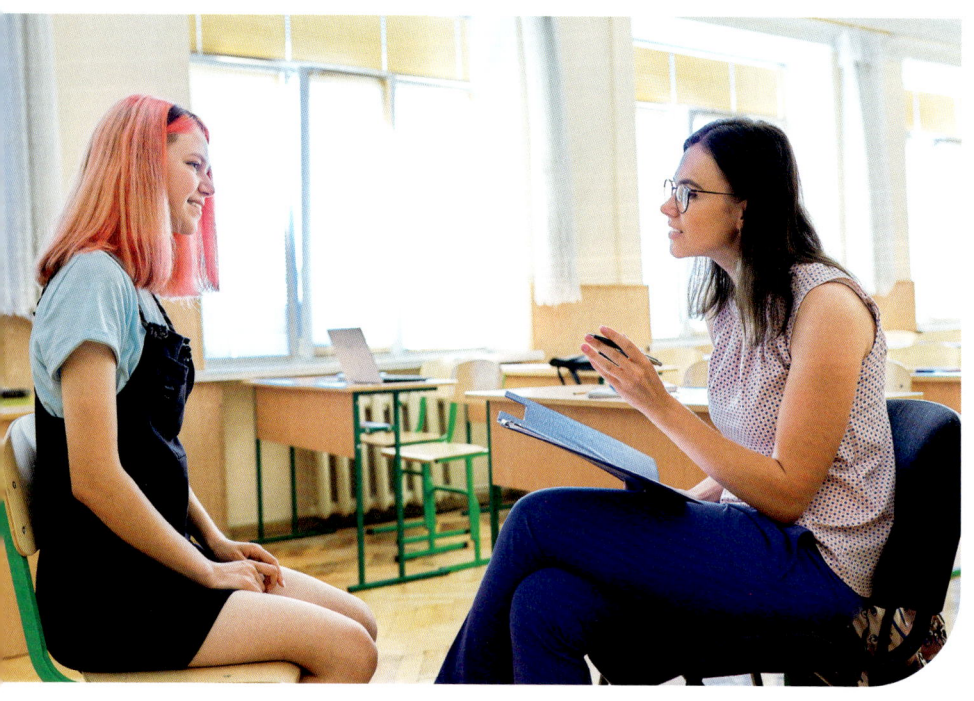

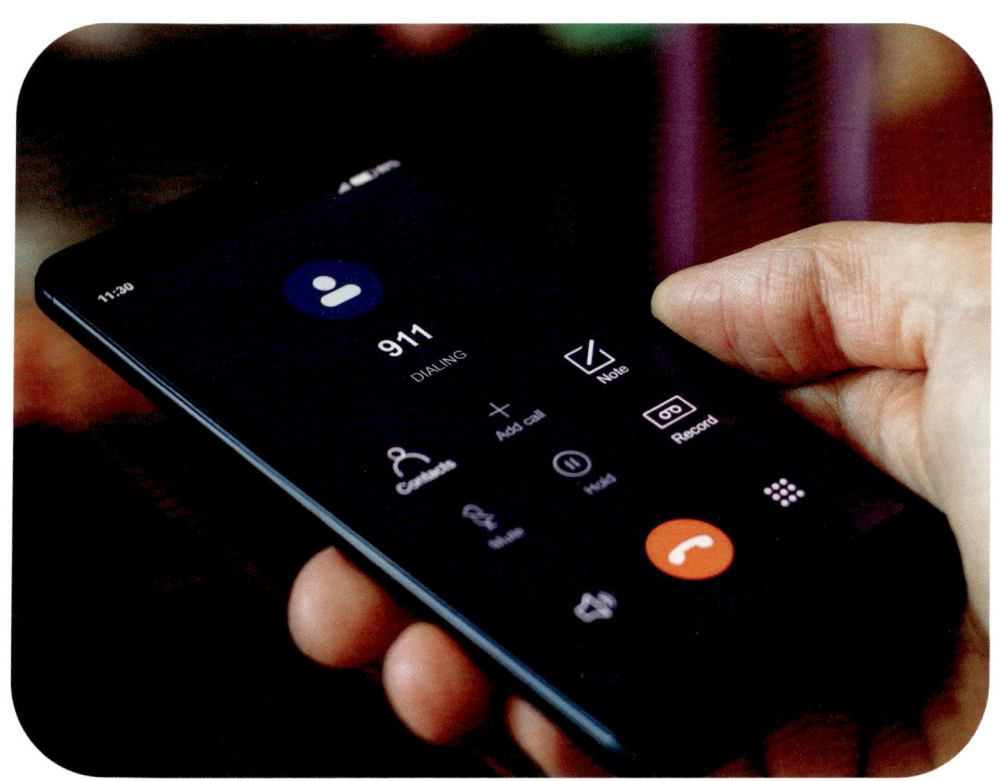

People should immediately call 911 if someone in crisis hurts themselves or attempts suicide.

Calling the police should be a last resort. Many mental health professionals believe the role of police should be reduced in mental health crisis situations. This is because people in crisis are often treated as criminals. However, the police are sometimes necessary if a weapon is involved.

CHAPTER THREE

LONG-TERM HELP AND HEALING

Parents, friends, and others can only help so much. Some people in crisis need professional help. They may need hospitalization or medication. Therapy could also be needed.

Schools often provide mental health services for students. Many schools have guidance counselors or psychologists. These professionals are available to talk to students. They can support those struggling

People should avoid being judgmental toward or blaming a person who is in crisis.

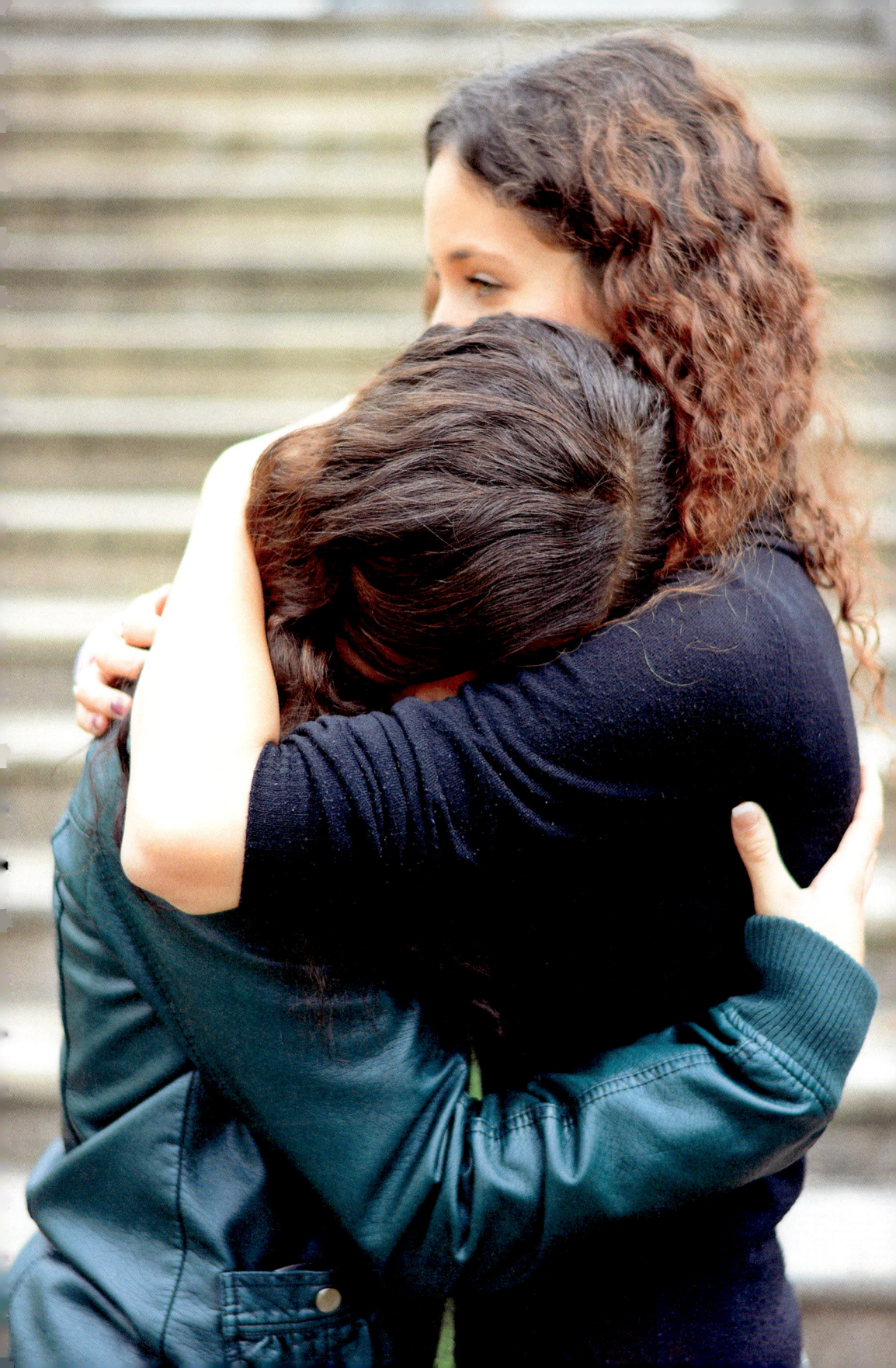

with mental health. They can also provide further resources if necessary.

Many communities provide mental health resources as well. Local programs and clinics can be found through

Psychologists can teach skills and techniques to help those in crisis better manage their mental health issues.

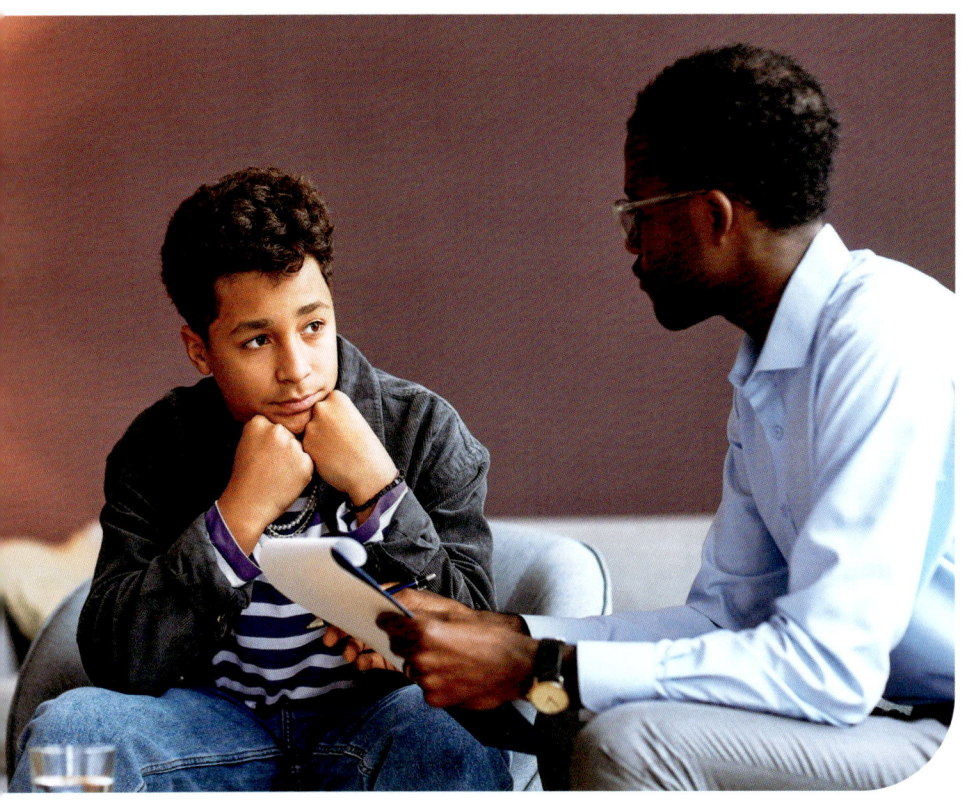

online searches. These places may offer appointments through call or text. Many places now have virtual appointments. Some clinics also take walk-ins.

For some people, an emergency room may be the first stop. "If you're not sure, go to the ER because we never want you to go without help," says child psychologist Jamie Becker. "But it's also important to know that the ER is not the only place that can help in a mental health crisis."[7]

Many communities have moved away from using police for mental health calls. Instead, some use Mobile Response Teams (MRTs). In Florida, people can call an MRT if they know or see someone in crisis. A team will go to wherever the person in crisis is. Trained staff arrive to diagnose problems.

They also know how to handle violent and dangerous situations.

CALL OR TEXT FOR HELP

Crisis hotlines are a key mental health resource. Suicide hotlines are especially important. Hotline staff listen and help people find the care they need. These hotlines are available every hour and every day of the year.

Different groups have special numbers to call. The suicide hotline number is 988. There are also numbers for LGBTQ+ teens, victims of abuse, and others dealing with trauma. Many hotlines help people calling on someone else's behalf.

Teen Line is a crisis hotline based in Los Angeles, California. It trains young

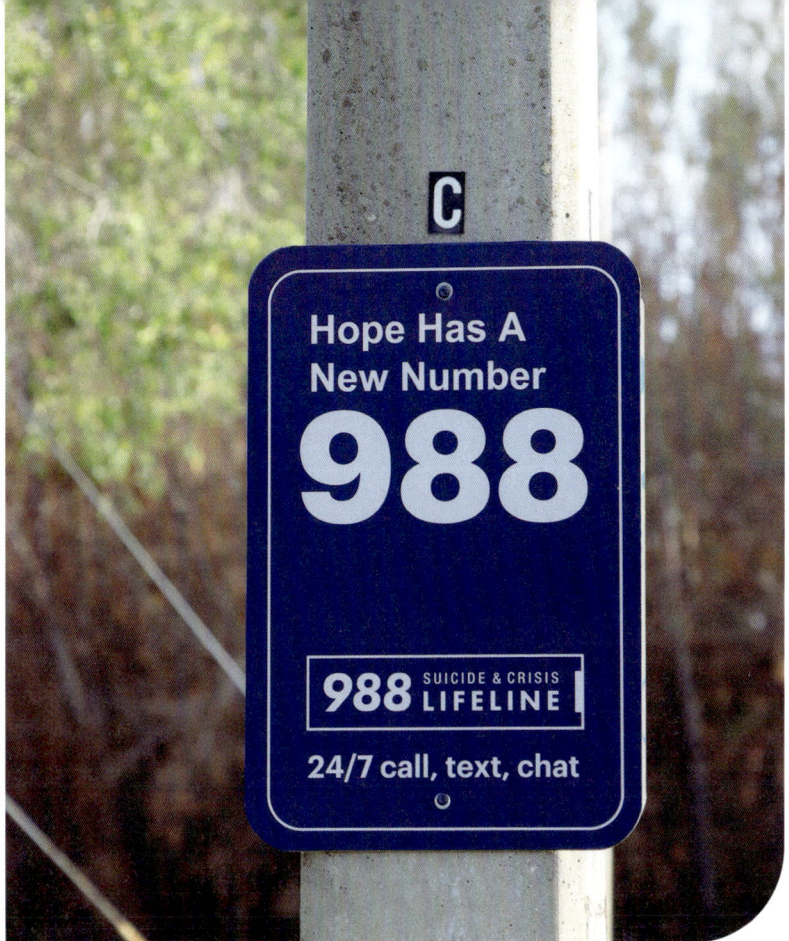

Most US states have started advertising the national suicide hotline number to bring more awareness to the resource.

operators on how to figure out whether callers are suicidal. In 2023, 16-year-old Mendez talked about her experiences as an operator. "People who are not suicidal will be like, 'No, no, no, no, I would never do that,'" she said. "But other people might say something like, 'Well, maybe . . . ' A lot of people will test the waters to make sure you're a safe person to tell."[8]

GETTING HELP ONLINE

Online resources have increased since 2020. This was mainly due to the COVID-19 pandemic. Today, some people in crisis access help online. Many sites make sure people's situations are anonymous and confidential.

After a crisis, some people need help from a therapist, psychologist, or psychiatrist. But booking appointments can be difficult. Many online resources are available. Some popular platforms include TalkSpace and Amwell. Pride Counseling provides therapy and counseling for

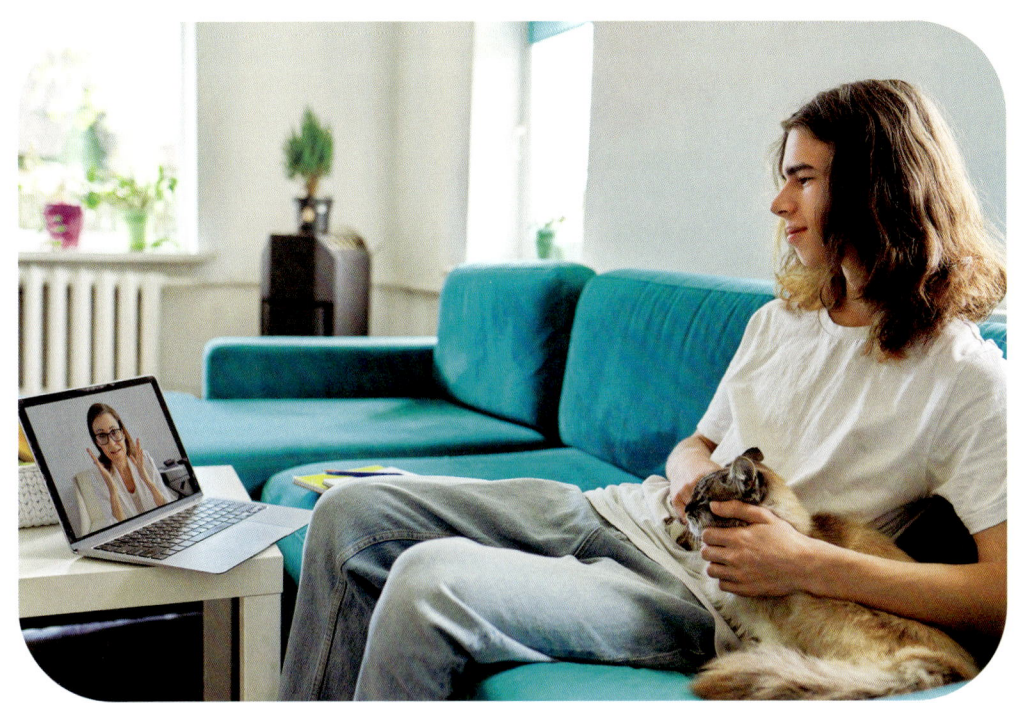

Some people feel more comfortable doing therapy sessions online rather than in person.

LGBTQ+ patients. Open Path Collective and other sites offer care as well.

Teens and adults will also turn to YouTube for support. Creators of all ages share their personal experiences online. They provide coping strategies. Many creators form communities around their channels. These communities help viewers feel less alone about their struggles.

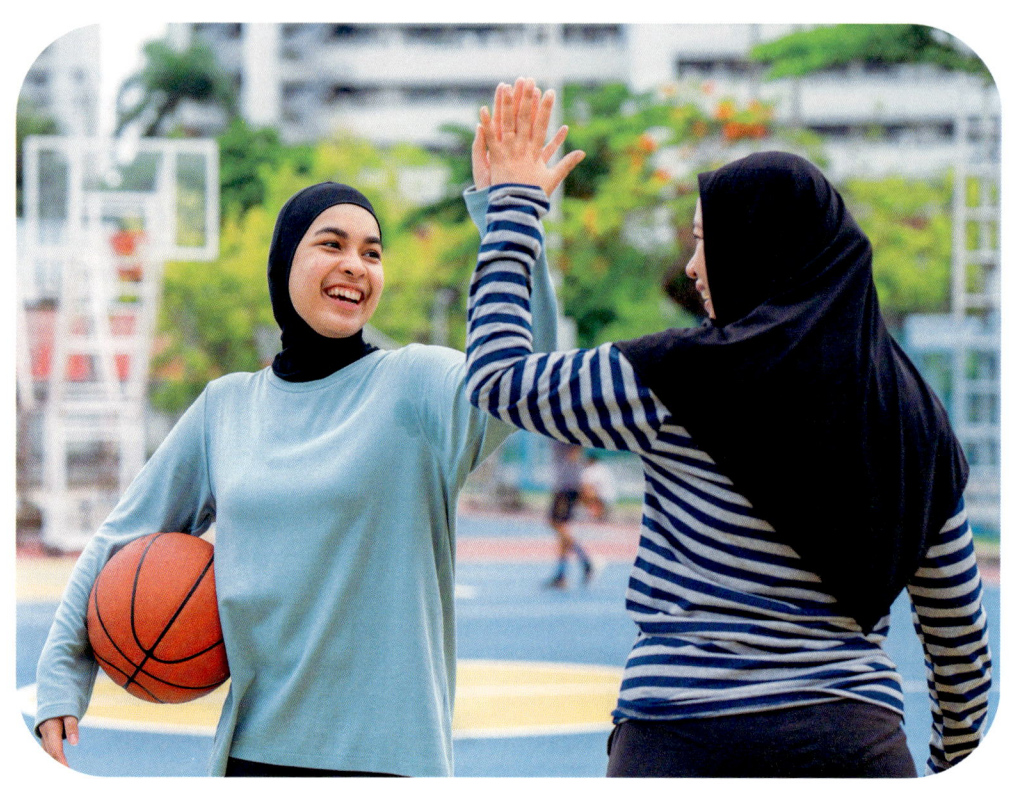

Self-care can include exercising regularly, eating healthy, setting goals, and focusing on positivity.

Finally, many phone apps are available as resources. Some examples include MindShift, HappiMe, Sanvello, and Woebot. The app MindShift encourages users to do a variety of tasks to improve their mental health. These include writing in journals, setting mental health goals, and practicing self-care.

SHARING STORIES AND STEPPING UP

The COVID-19 pandemic exposed a shortage of mental health professionals and facilities. Adults and youth both struggled to get therapy and support. Kids also suffered from being disconnected from one another.

Many schools and communities have taken action. They have launched programs where kids help others their age. Peer-to-peer counseling and meetups have become popular. Teens often feel more comfortable with their peers. Even caring adults can seem intimidating sometimes. Peer support can happen one-on-one, in groups, and in online chats.

Peer support is powerful. Both sides can benefit. Teens affected by mental health issues share similar experiences. They express their emotions and thoughts in a safe space. Teens who are helping can feel better about themselves too. They might feel as though they have a purpose. Helping peers can increase people's self-esteem and confidence.

LONG-TERM HEALING

Mental health issues can last weeks, months, or years. Long-term help is sometimes needed after a crisis. Psychologist Kenneth Carter writes, "Having someone around when you are going through a painful experience can be incredibly supportive. For **chronic** events like grief or long illnesses, it can be even more important in the weeks and months to come."[9]

Finola Summerville was very active in high school. She took the toughest courses, played sports, and volunteered. Finola also hid intense anxiety for years. This anxiety turned into depression. Eventually, the depression led to suicidal thoughts.

The Green Bandana Project

The Green Bandana Project is a school program working to reduce mental health crises. It also brings awareness to mental health issues. The program was inspired by Daniel Gerbec's story. Daniel died by suicide at age 14. He often wore a bandana. A green bandana became the symbol for the program. Green is the color for mental health awareness.

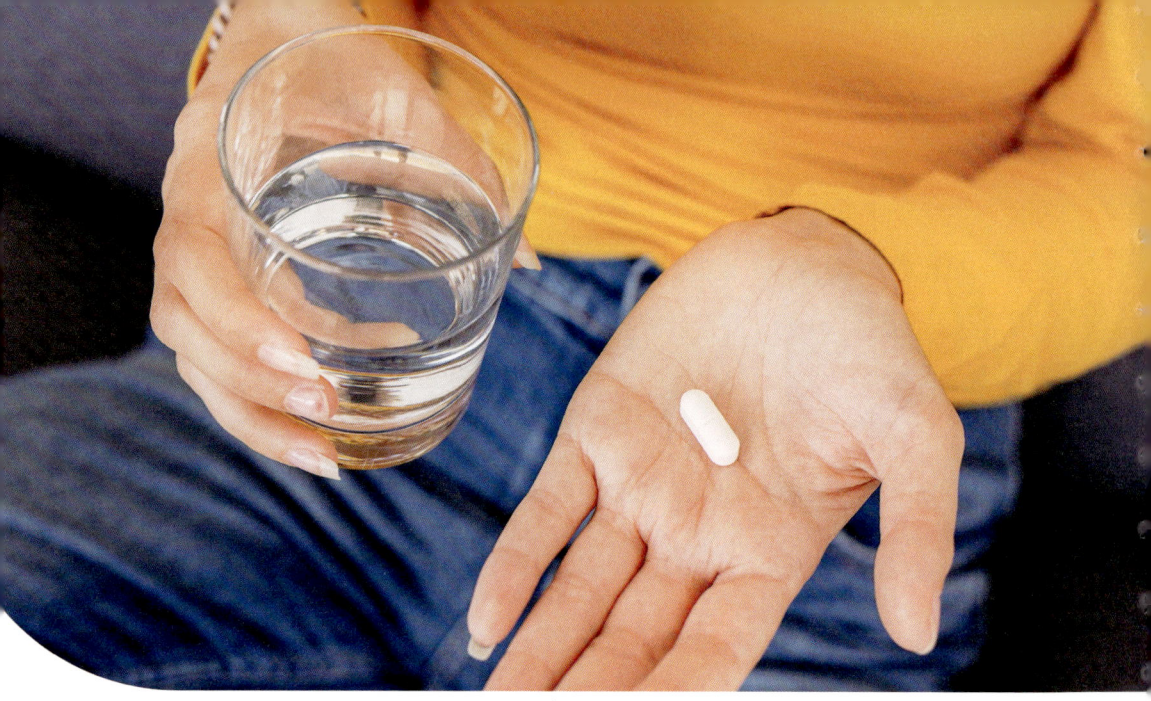

Some teens take medications to help manage their mental health struggles.

Finola finally spoke to an old friend about her thoughts. She was shocked to find out they also had suicidal feelings. The conversation inspired her. She decided it was time to get treatment. She saw a school social worker, went to therapy, and started medication.

Finola's school and community have also helped her heal. She found that help can sometimes come from unexpected places.

She began to understand that her mental health struggles were not something to be ashamed of.

SUPPORT THOSE IN CRISIS

Helping someone through a mental health crisis is just the start. Mental health

Support groups allow teens to talk to others who are dealing with similar problems.

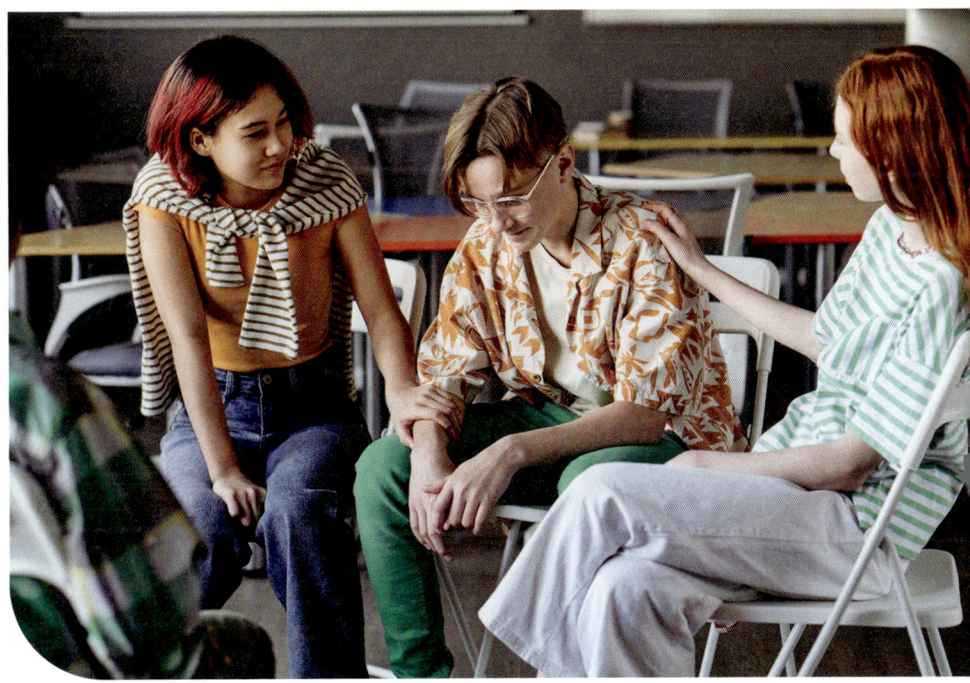

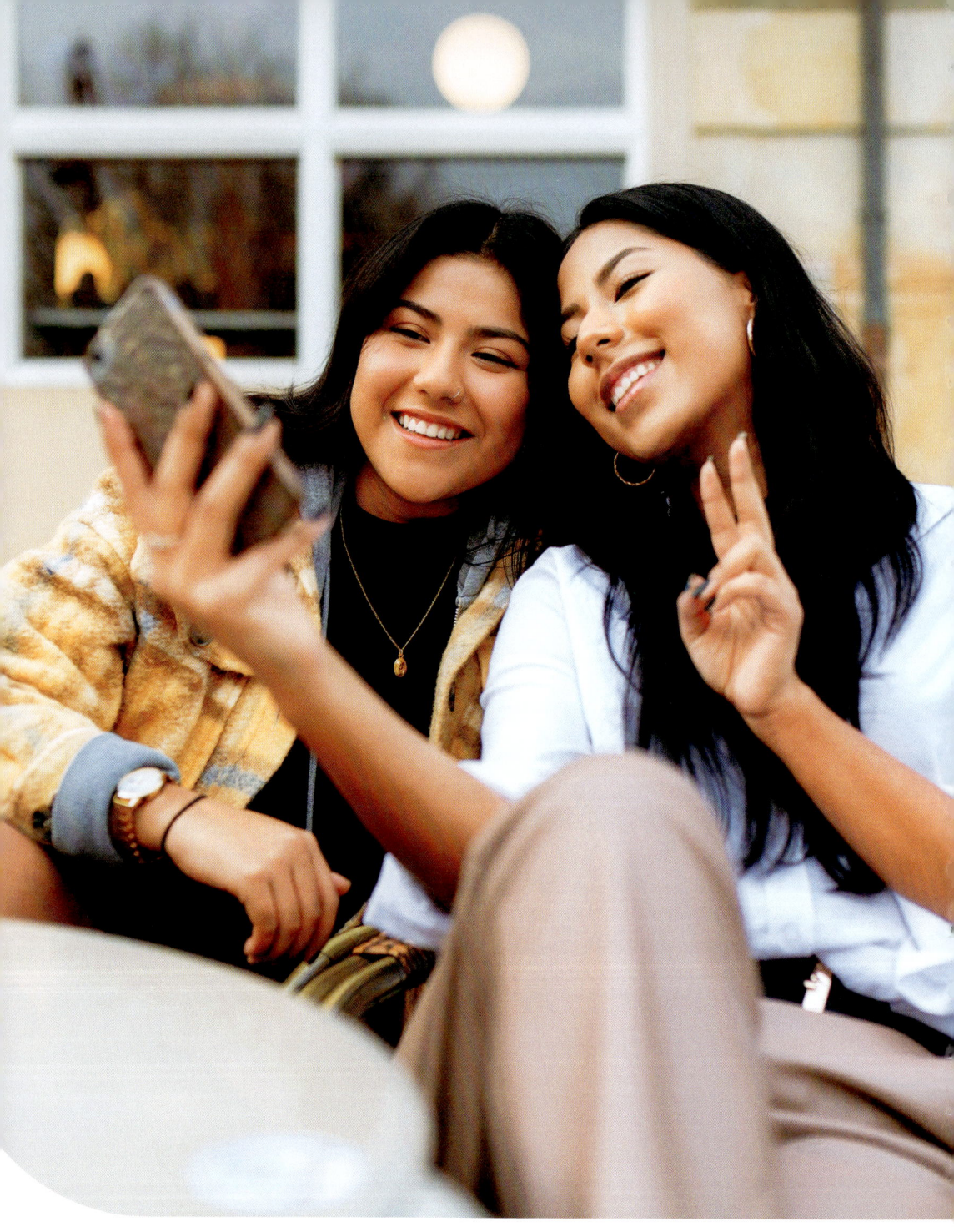

Providing support is an important part of helping teens overcome mental health crises.

struggles can last for years. This means people need long-term support. Family and friends can be a great support system. People can encourage those in crisis to continue their therapy appointments or take their medications. They can check in to see how the person feels. And they can recommend tools that help a particular mental health condition.

Friends can also volunteer to do things for their friends. These might include driving them to appointments. It could be helping with laundry or other tasks. Above all, being there is important. Including friends in plans and asking about their progress is also part of supporting them. Helping people through a crisis is the first step forward.

GLOSSARY

burnout

a state of mental, physical, and emotional tiredness caused by constant stress

chronic

something that persists for a long time, such as an illness

coping

managing negative thoughts and feelings to help deal with difficult life situations

empathy

the ability to understand and share the feelings of other people

marginalized

referring to people who are considered unimportant or less than by society

traumatic

emotionally or psychologically shocking or distressing

validated

having feelings or emotions that are acknowledged and supported by others

vent

to express a strong emotion

SOURCE NOTES

INTRODUCTION: FINDING WAYS TO HELP

1. Quoted in Madi Donham, "Teen Inspires Action for Mental Health After Helping Hundreds Through Crisis Line Volunteerism," *Points of Light*, May 29, 2023. www.pointsoflight.org.

CHAPTER ONE: IDENTIFYING A MENTAL HEALTH CRISIS

2. Sierra, "Sierra's Story," *National Alliance on Mental Illness*, August 2, 2016. www.nami.org.

3. Lisa Damour, "When Your Child's Friend Is in Crisis," *New York Times*, January 20, 2016. https://archive.nytimes.com.

CHAPTER TWO: ENGAGING SOMEONE IN CRISIS

4. Quoted in "Read Their Stories, Hear Their Words," *Denver Post*, n.d. https://youthsuicide.denverpost.com.

5. Kenneth Carter, "Friends in Crisis: What to Do When You Don't Know What to Do," *Psychology Today*, September 17, 2019. www.psychologytoday.com.

6. Quoted in Katherine Martinelli, "How to Support a Friend Who Is Struggling," *Child Mind Institute*, February 3, 2025. https://childmind.org.

CHAPTER THREE: LONG-TERM HELP AND HEALING

7. Quoted in "When Should I Take My Child to the ER for Mental Health?" *Children's Health*, n.d. www.childrens.com.

8. Quoted in Sonja Sharp, "He Died Training for L.A. Teen Crisis Hotline. His Parents Want All to Know the Number," *Los Angeles Times*, November 30, 2023. www.latimes.com.

9. Carter, "Friends in Crisis: What to Do When You Don't Know What to Do."

FOR FURTHER RESEARCH

BOOKS

Mary Bates, *Teen Guide: Depression*. BrightPoint Press, 2026.

Jill Keppeler, *Mental Health for All*. Rosen Publishing, 2021.

Sheryl Normandeau, *Living with Anxiety*. BrightPoint Press, 2024.

INTERNET SOURCES

"Mental Health by the Numbers," *National Alliance on Mental Illness*, April 2023. www.nami.org.

"Read Their Stories, Hear Their Words," *Denver Post*, n.d. https://youthsuicide.denverpost.com.

"Supporting Someone in a Crisis," *Eisenberg Family Depression Center*, n.d. https://depressioncenter.org.

WEBSITES

Mental Health America
https://mhanational.org

Mental Health America is a nonprofit organization dedicated to promoting mental health, well-being, and illness prevention. The site provides information to increase mental health awareness and includes ways for young people to get involved.

National Alliance on Mental Illness
www.nami.org

The National Alliance on Mental Illness (NAMI) is an organization focused on providing mental health support. The organization's website includes a list of warning signs and symptoms in both children and adults for a variety of mental illnesses.

Substance Abuse and Mental Health Services Administration
www.samhsa.gov

The Substance Abuse and Mental Health Services Administration (SAMHSA) is a US government agency working to improve mental health treatment, access, and education. The site offers resources, such as hotlines and programs, that can help people who are struggling with mental health.

INDEX

Anees, Azin, 6–9
anxiety, 14, 16, 17, 19–21, 33, 37, 53

bullying, 10, 16

Carter, Kenneth, 34, 52
coping, 35, 49
COVID-19 pandemic, 15, 48, 51

depression, 14, 16, 17, 19–21, 28, 53

engaging, 33–34

Green Bandana Project, 53

hospitals, 20, 42, 45
hotlines, 8, 46

LGBTQ+ teens, 18, 46, 49
listening, 8, 30, 32, 37, 46

Macchia, Lindsay, 38–39
marginalized groups, 18
medications, 42, 54, 57
mental health professionals, 39, 41, 42, 48, 51
Mobile Response Team (MRT), 45

peer counseling, 36, 51
physical abuse, 17, 38, 46
pressures, 15–16, 19

resources, 11, 36, 37, 44, 46, 48, 50

Samaritans, 6–8
Satterfield, Stephen, 31
schools, 8, 12, 16, 36, 39, 42, 51, 53, 54
self-care, 16, 25, 50
self-harm, 20, 25
social media, 12, 30
substance abuse, 10, 18, 23, 38
suicide, 6, 18, 26, 28–31, 46–47, 53–54
Summerville, Finola, 53–55
support, 10–11, 18, 22, 28, 33, 42, 49, 51–52, 55–57

therapy, 20, 42, 48, 51, 54, 57
Trevor Project, 18
trusted adults, 37, 39

warning signs, 11, 21–27

IMAGE CREDITS

Cover: © Photoroyalty/Shutterstock Images
5: © Egoitz Bengoetxea Iguaran/iStockphoto
7: © PeopleImages.com-Yuri A./Shutterstock Images
9: © sturti/iStockphoto
10: © Monkey Business Images/Shutterstock Images
11: © Lee Snider Photo Images/Shutterstock Images
13: © Lisa F. Young/Shutterstock Images
14: © pikselstock/Shutterstock Images
17: © Red Line Editorial
21: © Fluid Shutter/Shutterstock Images
23: © Victor Moussa/Shutterstock Images
24: © FollowTheFlow/iStockphoto
26: © SDI Productions/iStockphoto
29: © Tassii/iStockphoto
31: © Daniel Hoz/Shutterstock Images
32: © Prostock-Studio/Shutterstock Images
35: © Mangostar/Shutterstock Images
38: © Prasit Rodphan/Shutterstock Images
40: © VH-Studio/Shutterstock Images
41: © Skrypnykov Dmytro/Shutterstock Images
43: © DavidTB/Shutterstock Images
44: © SeventyFour/Shutterstock Images
47: © Deutschlandreform/Shutterstock Images
49: © VH-Studio/Shutterstock Images
50: © Kingmaya Studio/Shutterstock Images
54: © Xavier Lorenzo/Shutterstock Images
55: © Anna Stills/Shutterstock Images
56: © Alberto Menendez Cervero/Shutterstock Images

ABOUT THE AUTHOR

Philip Wolny is a writer, editor, and copy editor originally hailing from Bydgoszcz, Poland, and raised in the New York City boroughs of Queens and Brooklyn. He has since settled in central Florida with his wife and daughter.